BLOOD TYPE A FOOD LIST

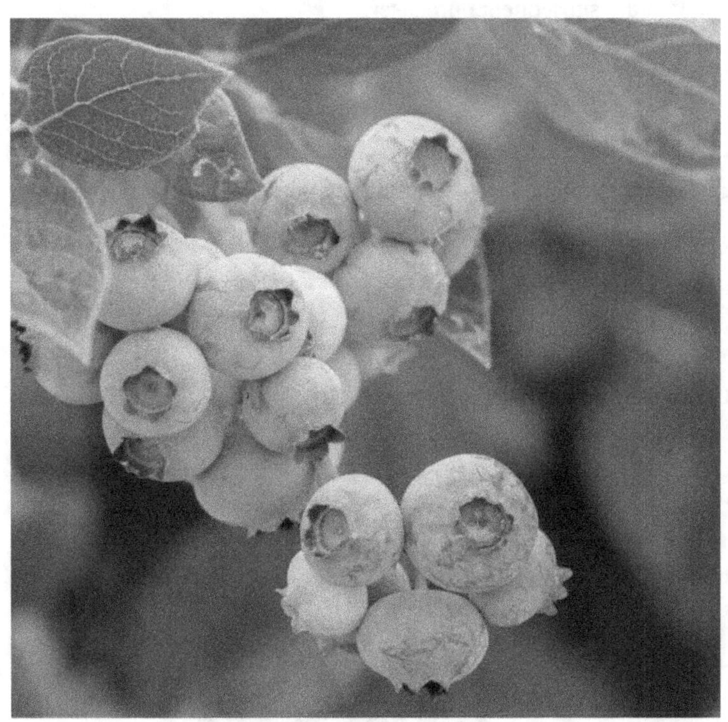

LORENE PEACHEY

Copyright © 2024 by Lorene Peachey

All rights reserved.

No part of this publication may be reproduced, stored in a retrieval system, or transmitted, in any form or by any means, electronic, mechanical, photocopying, recording or otherwise, without the prior written permission of the copyright holder.

This book is sold subject to the condition that it shall not, by way of trade or otherwise, be lent, re-sold, hired out or otherwise circulated without the publisher's prior consent in any form of binding or cover other than that in which it is published and without a similar condition including this condition being imposed on the subsequent purchaser.

DISCLAIMER

The content within this book reflects my thoughts, experiences, and beliefs. It is meant for informational and entertainment purposes. While I have taken great care to provide accurate information, I cannot guarantee the absolute correctness or applicability of the content to every individual or situation. Please consult with relevant professionals for advice specific to your needs.

TO GAIN ACCESS TO MORE BOOK BY THE AUTHOR SCAN THE QR CODE

TABLE OF CONTENTS

INTRODUCTION

In the delicate dance of life, food plays the lead role, determining the rhythm of our health and vitality. For me, Lorene Peachey, this symphony of sustenance has been my lifelong pursuit, a journey woven with passion, dedication, and a relentless quest for understanding the intimate connection between our blood types and the foods we consume. Allow me to share the heartwarming melody of my devotion to crafting extraordinary recipes tailored for Blood Type A.

Over the past 25 years, I've embarked on an odyssey through the realms of nutrition, delving deep into the intricate dance between blood types and dietary needs. My name is synonymous with a fervent commitment to unraveling the mysteries that lie within the very essence of our being, and it all began with a simple question that ignited a flame within me: What if our unique blood types held the key to unlocking a realm of well-being and health?

As a seasoned nutritionist, I've witnessed the transformative power of food in countless lives. Yet, it was the prospect of understanding how our blood types influence our dietary requirements that fueled my insatiable curiosity. In this quest, I have meticulously explored the intricacies of Blood Type A, delving into the profound impact that tailored nutrition can have on one's health and vitality.

Imagine a culinary journey where each dish is not just a delightful feast for the taste buds but a harmonious ode to your unique genetic makeup. It's more than a diet; it's a symphony of flavors and nutrients orchestrated to resonate with the very core of your being. Through years of research, I have carefully curated a food list specifically designed for Blood Type A individuals, blending science with creativity to craft meals that are not only delicious but also hold the key to unlocking the door to a healthier, more vibrant life.

The benefits of aligning your diet with your blood type are nothing short of extraordinary. Picture this: every bite you take is not just a source of nourishment; it's a personalized elixir tailored to enhance your well-being. But, dear reader, allow me to pose a question that stirs the emotions within: Have you ever wondered why a generic, one-size-fits-all approach to nutrition might not be yielding the results you desire?

Consider this: the consequences of neglecting your unique dietary needs could be far-reaching. It's not just about what you eat but understanding how your body responds to certain foods. Eating against the grain of your blood type can lead to a cacophony of health issues – from digestive woes to sluggishness that dulls the sparkle in your eyes. The symphony of life requires harmony, and what better way to achieve it than by savoring the foods that resonate with your very essence?

Herein lies the essence of my life's work – a culinary journey that transcends the mundane, a dance with flavors that syncs seamlessly with the rhythm of your health. The dangers of disregarding your blood type in your dietary choices could manifest in ways you least expect. It's not merely about what you see on the surface; it's about nurturing your body from within, setting the stage for a radiant, vibrant life.

As you explore the vibrant palette of Blood Type A-friendly foods, envision a life where every meal is a celebration of health. The advantage of having this meticulously crafted food list extends beyond the realm of physical health. It's an invitation to savor the joy of living fully, experiencing boundless energy, and relishing a sense of balance that emanates from within.

Now, let me take you by the hand and guide you through the tantalizing world of my culinary creations. Picture the aroma of a quinoa and vegetable stir-fry wafting through your kitchen, a melody of colors and flavors that not only delights your senses but also nourishes your body at its core. Or imagine the succulence of a baked salmon infused with the essence of lemon and herbs, a dish that not only tantalizes your taste buds but also provides your body with the omega-3 fatty acids it craves.

In this culinary journey, I've harnessed the power of nature's bounty to create recipes that not only align with your blood type but also elevate your overall well-being. From hearty lentil soups that warm your soul to vibrant berry smoothie bowls that awaken your senses – each dish is a testament to the art of living in harmony with your body's unique needs.

But, dear reader, the magic of this journey lies not just in the recipes but in the transformation they can bring to your life. It's about embracing the joy of conscious eating, where each morsel becomes a mindful step towards a healthier, happier you. As you peruse the pages of this culinary guide, I invite you to reflect on the connection between your blood type and the foods that grace your plate. Allow yourself to be captivated by the possibilities that await – a journey where every meal is a step towards optimal well-being and a life lived in full bloom.

So, let the adventure begin! Through the pages of this book, immerse yourself in the tantalizing world of Blood Type A-friendly recipes. Join me in savoring the flavors, unlocking the secrets, and relishing the transformative power of embracing a diet that resonates with your very essence. It's not just a book; it's a passport to a culinary voyage that holds the promise of a healthier, more vibrant you. Welcome to a world where the art of living meets the science of nutrition, and every meal is a celebration of life.

Contact the Author

Thank you for reading my book! I would love to hear from you, whether you have feedback, questions, or just want to share your thoughts. Your feedback means a lot to me and helps me improve as a writer.

Please don't hesitate to reach out to me through

lorenepeachey@gmail.com

I look forward to connecting with my readers and appreciate your support in this literary journey. Your thoughts and comments are valuable to me.

CHAPTER 1

OVERVIEW OF BLOOD TYPE A

Blood Type A is one of the four main blood types, characterized by the presence of A antigens on the surface of red blood cells. Individuals with Blood Type A often possess certain unique traits and characteristics. This blood type is believed to have originated in agrarian societies, and as a result, individuals with Blood Type A are thought to thrive on plant-based diets.

Characteristics of Blood Type A Individuals:

1. **Adaptability:** People with Blood Type A are often described as adaptable and cooperative. They may exhibit a sensitive and detail-oriented nature.

2. **Agrarian Heritage:** The theory suggests that Blood Type A may have evolved in response to the shift from hunting to agriculture, influencing the dietary needs of individuals with this blood type.

3. **Stress Sensitivity:** Blood Type A individuals may be more prone to stress, and it is believed that certain lifestyle and dietary choices can help manage stress levels effectively.

Importance of Blood Type in Diet

The concept of tailoring diets based on blood types gained popularity through the work of Dr. Peter J. D'Adamo, who proposed that individuals with different blood types have different nutritional needs. According to this theory, adhering to a diet aligned with one's blood type can promote overall well-being and reduce the risk of various health issues.

Key Points:

1. **Nutrient Absorption:** The idea is that certain blood types may have specific abilities or challenges in absorbing certain nutrients, influencing the types of foods that are beneficial or detrimental.

2. **Disease Prevention:** Advocates of blood type-based diets suggest that aligning one's diet with their blood type can contribute to disease prevention and improved health outcomes.

3. **Energy Levels:** Tailoring the diet to match the evolutionary history associated with a particular blood type is believed to optimize energy levels and support better digestion.

CHAPTER 2

BLOOD TYPE A

CHARACTERISTICS

Physical Traits:

1. **Moderate Build:** Individuals with Blood Type A typically have a moderate, balanced build.

2. **Agrarian Features:** There may be characteristics associated with agrarian ancestry, such as a tendency toward a well-functioning immune system and efficient digestive system.

3. **Sensitivity to Environmental Factors:** Blood Type A individuals might exhibit sensitivity to environmental factors, making them more adaptable to changes in diet and lifestyle.

Personality Traits:

1. **Adaptable:** Blood Type A personalities are often described as adaptable and cooperative. They tend to be flexible and able to adjust to various situations.

2. **Detail-Oriented:** People with Blood Type A may have a detail-oriented and analytical nature. They often pay attention to the finer points of situations.

3. **Reserved:** Blood Type A individuals may lean towards introversion and be reserved in social settings. They may value deeper, more meaningful connections.

Metabolic Considerations:

1. **Moderate Metabolism:** Blood Type A individuals are associated with a moderate metabolic rate, requiring a balanced approach to caloric intake.

2. **Stress Sensitivity:** There is a suggested sensitivity to stress, with stress management playing a crucial role in maintaining overall well-being.

Exercise Preferences:

1. **Calming Exercises:** Blood Type A individuals may benefit from exercises that promote relaxation and reduce stress, such as yoga, tai chi, or meditation.

2. **Routine and Consistency:** Establishing a consistent exercise routine can be beneficial for maintaining physical and mental balance.

Dietary Considerations:

1. **Plant-Based Emphasis:** Blood Type A is often linked to an agrarian history, and individuals with this blood type may thrive on a primarily plant-based diet.

2. **Lean Proteins:** While animal proteins are not entirely excluded, lean sources of protein such as fish and poultry are typically recommended over red meat.

3. **Avoidance of Certain Foods:** Blood Type A individuals may be advised to limit or avoid certain foods, such as dairy and red meat, to support optimal digestion and overall health.

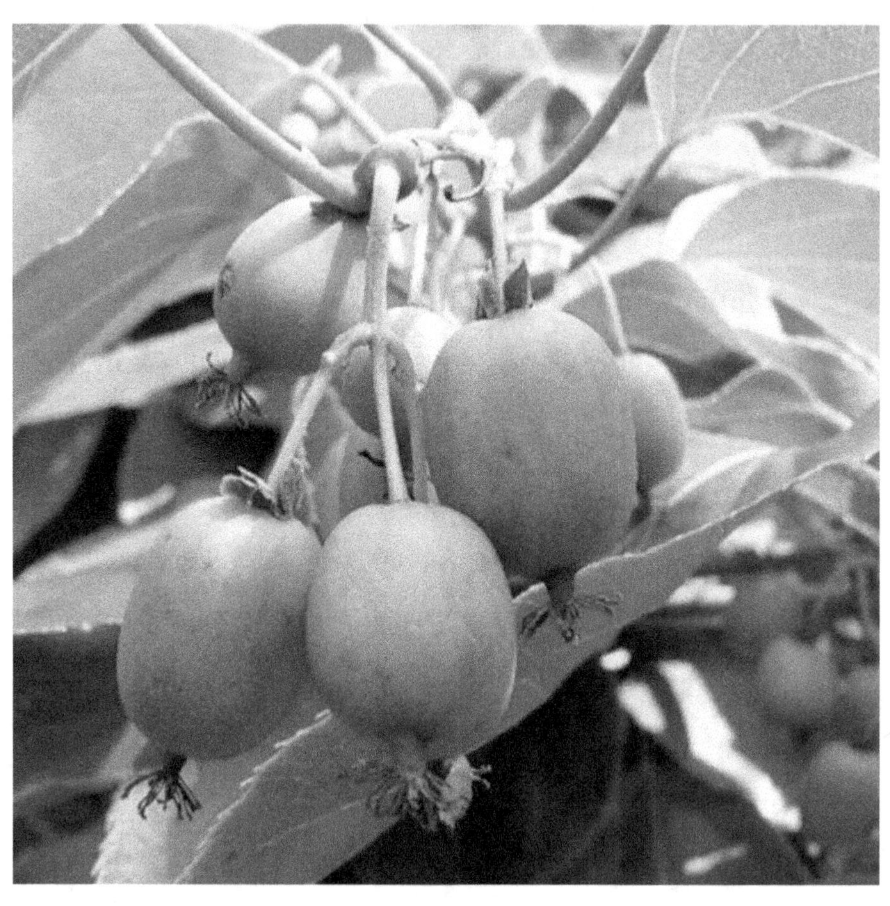

CHAPTER 3

FRUITS

1. **Blueberries:**

   - Nutritional Information (per 100g):

     - Calories: 57

     - Carbohydrates: 14.5g

     - Fiber: 2.4g

     - Vitamin C: 9.7mg

     - Antioxidants: Rich in anthocyanins, quercetin, and vitamin C.

2. **Apples:**

- Nutritional Information (medium-sized apple):

    - Calories: 95

    - Carbohydrates: 25g

    - Fiber: 4g

    - Vitamin C: 14% of the Daily Value (DV)

    - Antioxidants: Contains flavonoids and polyphenols.

3. **Pears:**

- Nutritional Information (medium-sized pear):

    - Calories: 101

    - Carbohydrates: 27g

    - Fiber: 6g

    - Vitamin C: 7% of the DV

    - Antioxidants: Rich in dietary fiber and flavonoids.

4. **Cherries:**

- Nutritional Information (per 100g):

    - Calories: 50

    - Carbohydrates: 12.2g

    - Fiber: 1.6g

    - Vitamin C: 7mg

    - Antioxidants: Contains anthocyanins and quercetin.

5. **Grapes:**

- Nutritional Information (per cup, about 151g):

    - Calories: 104

    - Carbohydrates: 27.3g

    - Fiber: 1.4g

    - Vitamin C: 4% of the DV

    - Antioxidants: Contains resveratrol and quercetin.

6. **Kiwi:**

- Nutritional Information (per medium-sized kiwi):

  - Calories: 61

  - Carbohydrates: 15g

  - Fiber: 2.1g

  - Vitamin C: 71% of the DV

  - Antioxidants: Rich in vitamin C and phytochemicals.

7. **Papaya:**

- Nutritional Information (per cup, about 145g):

  - Calories: 62

  - Carbohydrates: 15.9g

  - Fiber: 2.5g

  - Vitamin C: 88% of the DV

  - Antioxidants: Contains papain and beta-carotene.

8. **Plums:**

- Nutritional Information (per medium-sized plum):

  - Calories: 30

  - Carbohydrates: 8g

  - Fiber: 1.1g

  - Vitamin C: 10% of the DV

  - Antioxidants: Rich in anthocyanins and vitamin C.

9. **Watermelon:**

- Nutritional Information (per cup, about 152g):

  - Calories: 46

  - Carbohydrates: 11.5g

  - Fiber: 0.6g

  - Vitamin C: 13% of the DV

  - Antioxidants: Contains lycopene and vitamin A.

10. **Cranberries:**

- Nutritional Information (per cup, about 95g, raw):

  - Calories: 46

  - Carbohydrates: 12.2g

  - Fiber: 4.6g

  - Vitamin C: 16% of the DV

  - Antioxidants: Rich in proanthocyanidins.

CHAPTER 4

VEGETABLES

1. **Spinach:**

    - Nutritional Information (per cup, raw):

        - Calories: 7

        - Carbohydrates: 1.1g

        - Fiber: 0.7g

        - Vitamin A: 2813 IU (56% of the Daily Value)

        - Vitamin K: 145mcg (181% of the DV)

2. **Broccoli:**

    - Nutritional Information (per cup, chopped, raw):

        - Calories: 31

        - Carbohydrates: 6g

        - Fiber: 2.4g

        - Vitamin C: 81mg (135% of the DV)

        - Vitamin K: 101mcg (127% of the DV)

3. **Carrots:**

- Nutritional Information (per medium-sized carrot):

    - Calories: 25

    - Carbohydrates: 6g

    - Fiber: 2g

    - Vitamin A: 10191 IU (204% of the DV)

    - Vitamin K: 8mcg (10% of the DV)

4. **Kale:**

- Nutritional Information (per cup, chopped, raw):

    - Calories: 33

    - Carbohydrates: 6.7g

    - Fiber: 1.3g

    - Vitamin A: 10302 IU (206% of the DV)

    - Vitamin K: 547mcg (684% of the DV)

5. **Sweet Potatoes:**

- Nutritional Information (medium-sized sweet potato, baked):

    - Calories: 103

    - Carbohydrates: 24g

    - Fiber: 3.8g

    - Vitamin A: 43858 IU (877% of the DV)

    - Vitamin C: 22.3mg (37% of the DV)

6. **Bell Peppers (Red):**

- Nutritional Information (per cup, chopped, raw):

    - Calories: 46

    - Carbohydrates: 9g

    - Fiber: 3g

    - Vitamin A: 3726 IU (75% of the DV)

    - Vitamin C: 190mg (317% of the DV)

7. **Cauliflower:**

- Nutritional Information (per cup, chopped, raw):

    - Calories: 27

    - Carbohydrates: 5.3g

    - Fiber: 2.5g

    - Vitamin C: 51.6mg (86% of the DV)

    - Vitamin K: 16mcg (20% of the DV)

8. **Cucumbers:**

- Nutritional Information (per cup, sliced, raw):

    - Calories: 16

    - Carbohydrates: 3.8g

    - Fiber: 0.5g

    - Vitamin K: 8.5mcg (11% of the DV)

    - Vitamin C: 2.8mg (5% of the DV)

9. **Zucchini:**

- Nutritional Information (per cup, sliced, raw):

    - Calories: 20

    - Carbohydrates: 4.1g

    - Fiber: 1.3g

    - Vitamin C: 21mg (35% of the DV)

    - Vitamin K: 7mcg (9% of the DV)

10. **Brussels Sprouts:**

- Nutritional Information (per cup, chopped, raw):

    - Calories: 38

    - Carbohydrates: 8g

    - Fiber: 3.3g

    - Vitamin C: 74.8mg (125% of the DV)

    - Vitamin K: 156mcg (195% of the DV)

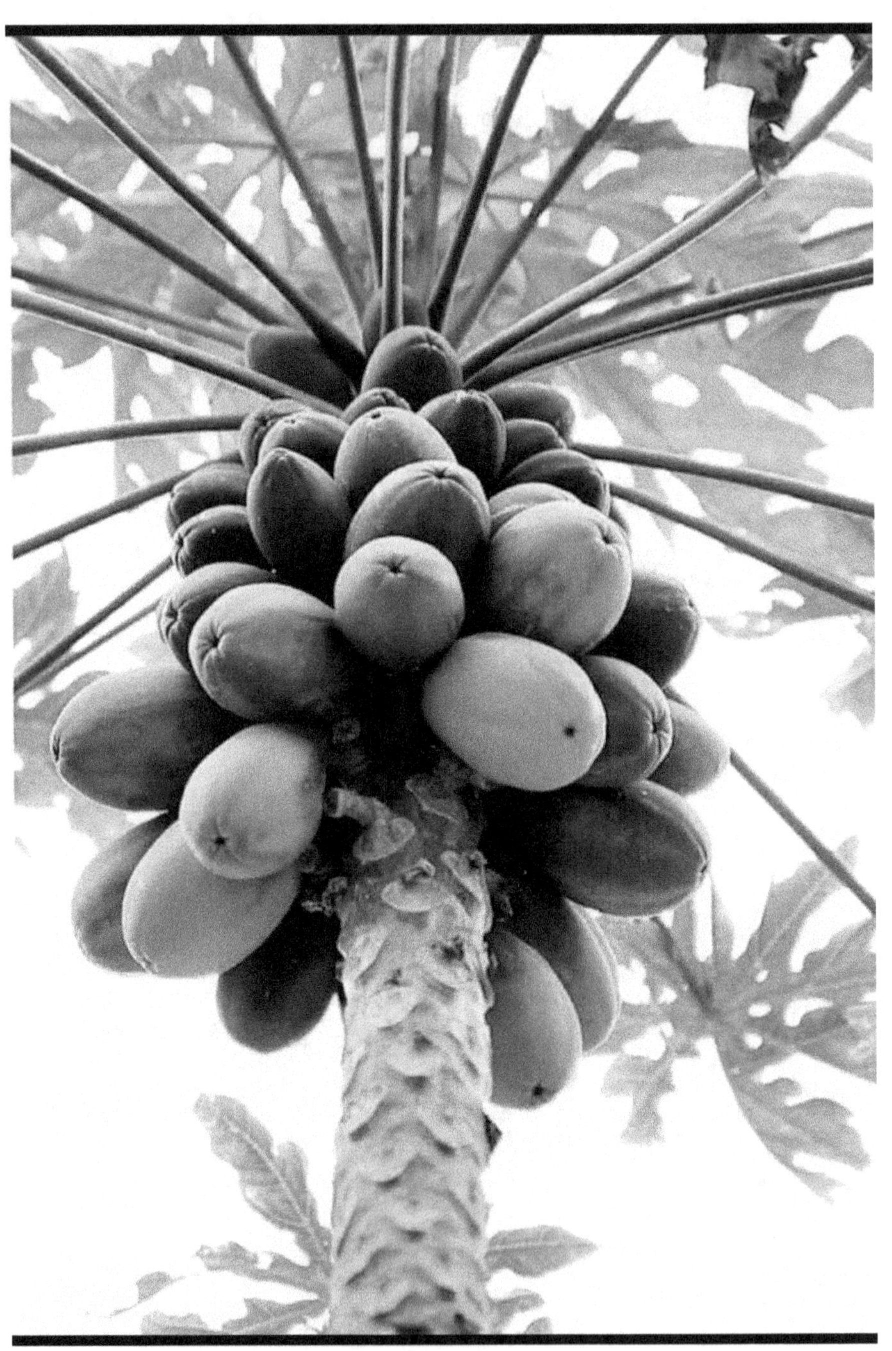

CHAPTER 5

PROTEIN SOURCES

1. **Salmon:**

    - Nutritional Information (per 3 oz, cooked):

        - Calories: 175

        - Protein: 23g

        - Omega-3 Fatty Acids: 1.6g

        - Vitamin D: 570 IU (142% of the Daily Value)

        - Selenium: 27mcg (39% of the DV)

2. **Tofu:**

    - Nutritional Information (per 1/2 cup, firm):

        - Calories: 94

        - Protein: 10g

        - Calcium: 404mg (40% of the DV)

        - Iron: 2.3mg (13% of the DV)

3. **Quinoa:**

- Nutritional Information (per 1 cup, cooked):

    - Calories: 222

    - Protein: 8g

    - Fiber: 5g

    - Iron: 2.8mg (15% of the DV)

    - Magnesium: 118mg (30% of the DV)

4. **Lentils:**

- Nutritional Information (per 1 cup, cooked):

    - Calories: 230

    - Protein: 18g

    - Fiber: 16g

    - Iron: 6.6mg (37% of the DV)

    - Folate: 358mcg (90% of the DV)

5. **Turkey (Lean Ground):**

- Nutritional Information (per 3 oz, cooked):

    - Calories: 135

    - Protein: 22g

    - Selenium: 25mcg (36% of the DV)

    - Zinc: 2.3mg (16% of the DV)

6. **Edamame:**

- Nutritional Information (per 1 cup, cooked):

    - Calories: 189

    - Protein: 17g

    - Fiber: 8g

    - Folate: 121mcg (30% of the DV)

    - Vitamin K: 52mcg (66% of the DV)

7. **Eggs:**

- Nutritional Information (per large egg, boiled):

    - Calories: 68

    - Protein: 6g

    - Vitamin B12: 0.6mcg (11% of the DV)

    - Selenium: 15.4mcg (22% of the DV)

8. **Soy Milk:**

- Nutritional Information (per 1 cup):

    - Calories: 80

    - Protein: 7g

    - Calcium: 301mg (23% of the DV)

    - Vitamin D: 2.9mcg (15% of the DV)

9. **Chickpeas (Garbanzo Beans):**

- Nutritional Information (per 1 cup, cooked):

    - Calories: 269

    - Protein: 14.5g

    - Fiber: 12.5g

    - Folate: 282mcg (71% of the DV)

    - Iron: 4.7mg (26% of the DV)

10. **Almonds:**

- Nutritional Information (per 1 oz, dry-roasted):

    - Calories: 170

    - Protein: 6g

    - Fiber: 3.5g

    - Vitamin E: 7.3mg (37% of the DV)

    - Magnesium: 76mg (19% of the DV)

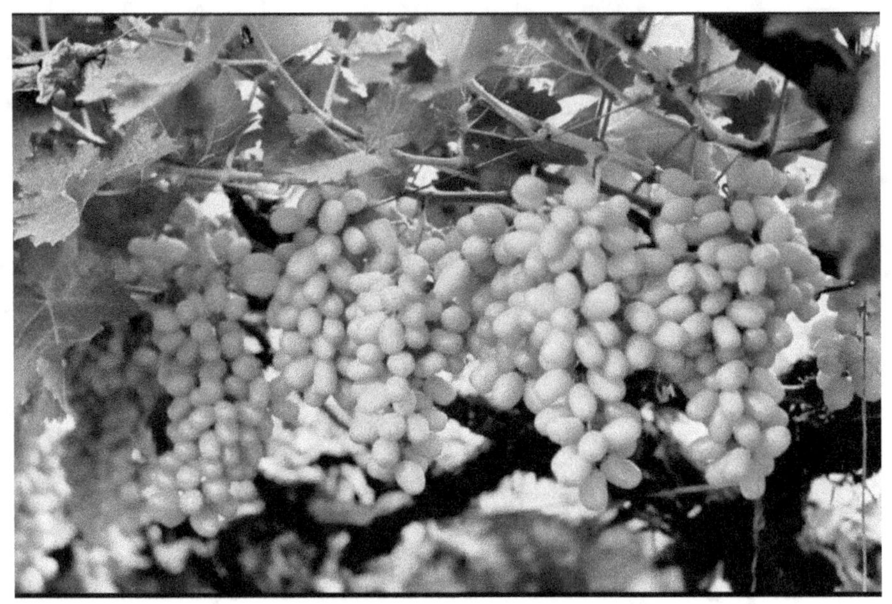

CHAPTER 6

GRAINS

1. **Quinoa:**

   - Nutritional Information (per 1 cup, cooked):

     - Calories: 222

     - Protein: 8g

     - Fiber: 5g

     - Iron: 2.8mg (15% of the Daily Value)

     - Magnesium: 118mg (30% of the DV)

2. **Brown Rice:**

   - Nutritional Information (per 1 cup, cooked):

     - Calories: 215

     - Protein: 5g

     - Fiber: 4g

     - Manganese: 1.8mg (88% of the DV)

     - Selenium: 19.1mcg (27% of the DV)

3. **Oats:**

- Nutritional Information (per 1 cup, cooked):

    - Calories: 147

    - Protein: 6g

    - Fiber: 4g

    - Manganese: 0.6mg (29% of the DV)

    - Phosphorus: 180mg (18% of the DV)

4. **Amaranth:**

- Nutritional Information (per 1 cup, cooked):

    - Calories: 251

    - Protein: 9g

    - Fiber: 5g

    - Calcium: 116mg (12% of the DV)

    - Iron: 5.2mg (29% of the DV)

5. **Buckwheat:**

- Nutritional Information (per 1 cup, cooked):

  - Calories: 155

  - Protein: 6g

  - Fiber: 5g

  - Manganese: 1.1mg (54% of the DV)

  - Magnesium: 86mg (21% of the DV)

6. **Millet:**

- Nutritional Information (per 1 cup, cooked):

  - Calories: 207

  - Protein: 6g

  - Fiber: 2g

  - Magnesium: 76mg (19% of the DV)

  - Phosphorus: 129mg (13% of the DV)

7. **Barley:**

- Nutritional Information (per 1 cup, cooked):

    - Calories: 193

    - Protein: 3.5g

    - Fiber: 6g

    - Manganese: 0.7mg (33% of the DV)

    - Selenium: 11.1mcg (16% of the DV)

8. **Spelt:**

- Nutritional Information (per 1 cup, cooked):

    - Calories: 246

    - Protein: 10.7g

    - Fiber: 7.6g

    - Phosphorus: 222mg (22% of the DV)

    - Manganese: 1.9mg (97% of the DV)

9. **Wild Rice:**

- Nutritional Information (per 1 cup, cooked):

  - Calories: 166

  - Protein: 6.5g

  - Fiber: 3g

  - Manganese: 1mg (51% of the DV)

  - Magnesium: 52mg (13% of the DV)

10. **Farro:**

- Nutritional Information (per 1 cup, cooked):

  - Calories: 220

  - Protein: 8g

  - Fiber: 8g

  - Magnesium: 68mg (17% of the DV)

  - Phosphorus: 313mg (31% of the DV)

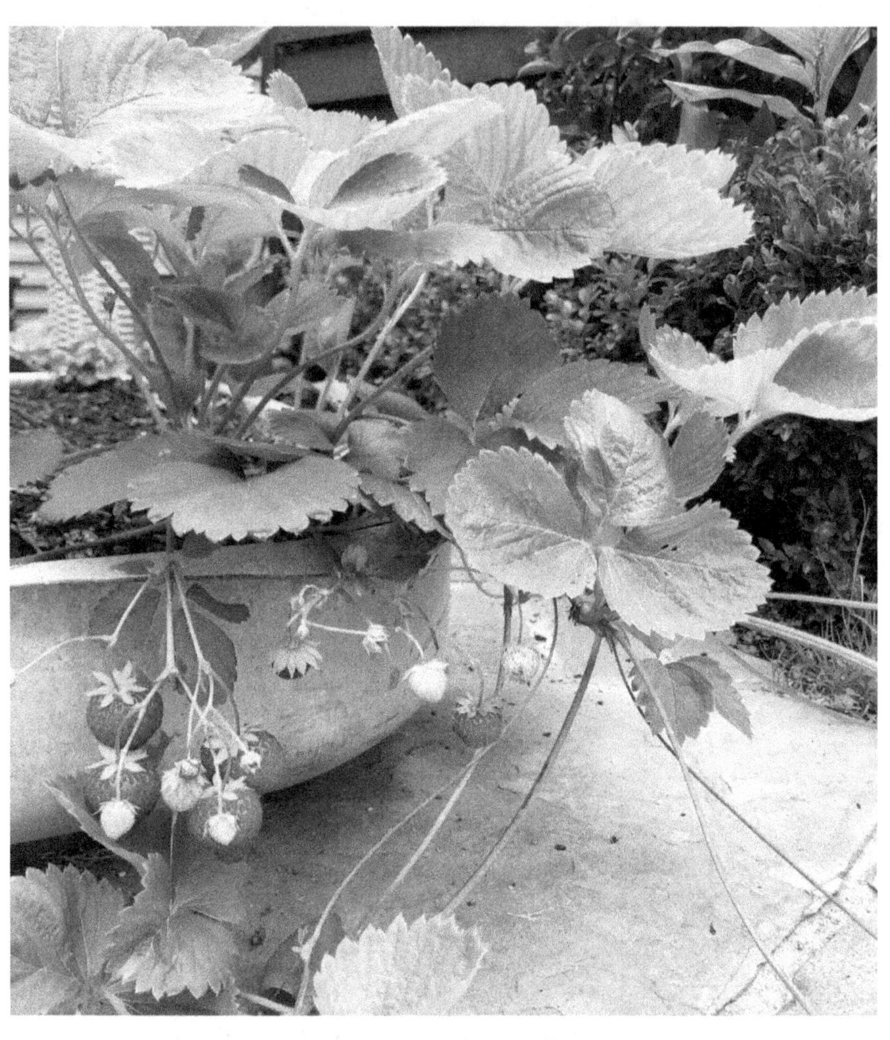

CHAPTER 7

FOODS TO AVOID

1. **Red Meat (Beef, Lamb):**

   - Nutritional Information (per 3 oz, cooked beef):

     - Calories: 250

     - Protein: 26g

     - Total Fat: 17g

     - Saturated Fat: 7g

     - Cholesterol: 94mg

2. **Dairy (Cow's Milk, Cheese):**

   - Nutritional Information (per 1 cup, whole milk):

     - Calories: 149

     - Protein: 7.7g

     - Total Fat: 7.9g

     - Saturated Fat: 4.6g

     - Cholesterol: 24mg

3. **Wheat-based Products:**

- Nutritional Information (per slice of white bread):

    - Calories: 79

    - Protein: 2.1g

    - Total Fat: 0.8g

    - Carbohydrates: 15.2g

4. **Tomatoes:**

- Nutritional Information (per medium-sized tomato):

    - Calories: 22

    - Protein: 1g

    - Total Fat: 0.2g

    - Carbohydrates: 5g

5. **Bananas:**

- Nutritional Information (per medium-sized banana):

    - Calories: 105

    - Protein: 1.3g

    - Total Fat: 0.3g

    - Carbohydrates: 27g

6. **Corn:**

- Nutritional Information (per cup, cooked):

    - Calories: 143

    - Protein: 5g

    - Total Fat: 2.7g

    - Carbohydrates: 31g

7. **Shellfish (Shrimp, Lobster):**

- Nutritional Information (per 3 oz, cooked shrimp):

    - Calories: 84

    - Protein: 18g

    - Total Fat: 1.5g

    - Cholesterol: 129mg

8. **Peanuts:**

- Nutritional Information (per 1 oz):

    - Calories: 161

    - Protein: 7.3g

    - Total Fat: 14g

    - Carbohydrates: 4.6g

9. **Avocado:**

- Nutritional Information (per medium-sized avocado):

    - Calories: 234

    - Protein: 3g

    - Total Fat: 21.4g

    - Carbohydrates: 12g

10. **Oranges:**

- Nutritional Information (per medium-sized orange):

    - Calories: 62

    - Protein: 1.2g

    - Total Fat: 0.2g

    - Carbohydrates: 15.4g

CHAPTER 8

GROCERY SHOPPING GUIDE

Embarking on a grocery shopping journey tailored to your Blood Type A can contribute to a balanced and potentially beneficial diet. While the Blood Type Diet is not universally supported by scientific evidence, if you choose to follow it, here's a guide to help you navigate the aisles:

1. Fresh Fruits:

- **Selection:** Opt for a variety of fruits rich in antioxidants and vitamins.

- **Examples:** Blueberries, apples, pears, cherries, kiwi, and cranberries.

- **Tip:** Choose organic options when possible to reduce exposure to pesticides.

2. Vegetables:

- **Selection:** Focus on a mix of colorful and leafy vegetables for a broad spectrum of nutrients.

- **Examples:** Spinach, broccoli, carrots, kale, sweet potatoes, and Brussels sprouts.

- **Tip:** Experiment with both raw and cooked vegetables to maximize nutritional benefits.

3. Lean Proteins:

- **Selection:** Choose lean protein sources to support your moderate metabolic rate.

- **Examples:** Salmon, tofu, lentils, turkey (lean ground), edamame, and eggs.

- **Tip:** Incorporate a variety of plant-based and animal-based proteins for a balanced approach.

4. Whole Grains:

- **Selection:** Opt for whole grains to provide essential carbohydrates and fiber.

- **Examples:** Quinoa, brown rice, oats, amaranth, buckwheat, and millet.

- **Tip:** Check labels for 100% whole grains to ensure maximum nutritional benefits.

5. Dairy Alternatives:

- **Selection:** Explore non-dairy alternatives for calcium and vitamin D.

- **Examples:** Soy milk and almond milk.

- **Tip:** Choose fortified options to supplement nutrients found in traditional dairy.

6. Nuts and Seeds:

- **Selection:** Include nuts and seeds for healthy fats and additional protein.

- **Examples:** Almonds and chia seeds.

- **Tip:** Consume in moderation; these can be great snacks or additions to meals.

7. Herbs and Spices:

- **Selection:** Enhance flavors without added salt by using herbs and spices.

- **Examples:** Turmeric, ginger, basil, and rosemary.

- **Tip:** Experiment with different combinations to keep your meals interesting.

8. Beverages:

- **Selection:** Stay hydrated with water, and explore herbal teas.

- **Examples:** Green tea and chamomile tea.

- **Tip:** Minimize sugary drinks and focus on hydrating, antioxidant-rich options.

9. Avoid or Limit:

- **Red Meat and Dairy:** Consider alternatives such as lean proteins and non-dairy options.

- **Wheat-based Products:** Choose gluten-free options like quinoa and rice.

- **Highly Processed Foods:** Opt for whole, minimally processed foods whenever possible.

10. Meal Planning:

- **Plan Ahead:** Prepare meals in advance to ensure a well-balanced diet.

- **Variety:** Embrace a variety of foods to maximize nutrient intake.

- **Listen to Your Body:** Pay attention to how your body responds to different foods.

IF YOU WANT MORE RECIPES, YOU CAN CHECK OUT OTHER BOOKS BY THE AUTHOR

GLUTEN-FREE COOKBOOK FOR MEN

GLUTEN-FREE COOKBOOK FOR WOMEN

GLUTEN-FREE COOKBOOK FOR SENIORS

MEDITERRANEAN SLOW COOKER COOKBOOK FOR WOMEN

LOW SODIUM COOKBOOK FOR SENIORS

TO GET ACCESS TO MORE BOOKS BY THE AUTHOR SCAN THE QR CODE

CONCLUSION

In closing this culinary journey tailored for Blood Type A, I am filled with gratitude for the opportunity to share my passion, knowledge, and recipes with you, dear reader. As we part ways, I invite you to reflect on the flavors, the nourishment, and the wellness woven into the fabric of this book.

The symphony of Blood Type A-friendly recipes presented here is not just a compilation of ingredients and instructions but a heartfelt offering designed to enrich your life. Each dish is a celebration of your unique genetic makeup, an ode to the harmonious connection between your blood type and the foods you consume.

Remember that this journey is not about rigid rules but an exploration of what truly nourishes your body, mind, and spirit. I encourage you to embrace the joy of conscious eating – savoring each bite, relishing the vibrant colors on your plate, and appreciating the nourishment that these recipes bring.

As you embark on incorporating these Blood Type A-friendly recipes into your life, I am eager to hear about your experiences, discoveries, and any culinary adventures you undertake. Your feedback is not just welcomed; it's an essential part of this ongoing dialogue. Share your insights, your favorite recipes, and even the challenges you faced. Your input contributes to the evolving tapestry of knowledge, fostering a community of individuals committed to optimal well-being through mindful nutrition.

In the spirit of continuous improvement, I invite you to reach out with your thoughts, questions, or even suggestions for future editions. Your feedback shapes the narrative of this culinary exploration and inspires the creation of even more delightful recipes crafted with your unique needs in mind.

Thank you for joining me on this enriching journey. May these recipes bring not only a symphony of flavors to your table but also a renewed sense of vitality, balance, and joy to your life. Here's to health, happiness, and the artistry of mindful eating!

BONUS CHAPTER 1

HEALTHY BLOOD TYPE A

RECIPES

Quinoa Salad with Mixed Vegetables

- **Cooking Time:** 20 minutes

- **Servings:** 4

Ingredients:

- 1 cup quinoa, rinsed

- 2 cups mixed vegetables (broccoli, bell peppers, cherry tomatoes)

- 1/4 cup feta cheese (optional)

- 2 tablespoons olive oil

- 1 tablespoon lemon juice

- Salt and pepper to taste

Instructions:

1. Cook quinoa according to package instructions.

2. Steam or lightly sauté mixed vegetables.

3. In a bowl, mix cooked quinoa, vegetables, feta cheese, olive oil, and lemon juice.

4. Season with salt and pepper.

5. Serve chilled.

Nutritional Information:

Per serving: Calories 280, Protein 8g, Fiber 6g, Healthy Fats 10g

Baked Salmon with Lemon and Herbs

- **Cooking Time:** 25 minutes

- **Servings:** 2

Ingredients:

- 2 salmon fillets

- 1 lemon, sliced

- 2 tablespoons olive oil

- 1 teaspoon dried herbs (such as thyme or dill)

- Salt and pepper to taste

Instructions:

1. Preheat oven to 375°F (190°C).

2. Place salmon fillets on a baking sheet.

3. Drizzle with olive oil and sprinkle with herbs, salt, and pepper.

4. Top with lemon slices.

5. Bake for 20-25 minutes until salmon is cooked through.

Nutritional Information:

Per serving: Calories 320, Protein 25g, Omega-3 Fatty Acids 1.5g

Stir-Fried Tofu with Vegetables

- **Cooking Time:** 15 minutes

- **Servings:** 3

Ingredients:

- 1 block firm tofu, cubed

- 2 cups mixed stir-fry vegetables (broccoli, snap peas, carrots)

- 3 tablespoons soy sauce

- 1 tablespoon sesame oil

- 1 teaspoon ginger, minced

Instructions:

1. Heat sesame oil in a pan, add tofu cubes, and stir-fry until golden.

2. Add vegetables and ginger, continue stirring.

3. Pour soy sauce over the mixture and cook until vegetables are tender.

Nutritional Information:

Per serving: Calories 250, Protein 15g, Fiber 4g

Millet and Vegetable Stuffed Peppers

- **Cooking Time:** 40 minutes

- **Servings:** 4

Ingredients:

- 1 cup millet, cooked

- 4 bell peppers, halved

- 1 cup black beans, cooked

- 1 cup corn kernels

- 1 cup diced tomatoes

- 1 teaspoon cumin

Instructions:

1. Preheat oven to 375°F (190°C).

2. In a bowl, mix cooked millet, black beans, corn, tomatoes, cumin, salt, and pepper.

3. Stuff bell peppers with the mixture.

4. Bake for 30 minutes or until peppers are tender.

Nutritional Information:

Per serving: Calories 280, Protein 10g, Fiber 8g

Turkey and Vegetable Stir-Fry

- **Cooking Time:** 20 minutes

- **Servings:** 4

Ingredients:

- 1 lb ground turkey

- 3 cups mixed stir-fry vegetables (bell peppers, broccoli, carrots)

- 2 tablespoons low-sodium soy sauce

- 1 tablespoon sesame oil

- 1 teaspoon garlic, minced

Instructions:

1. In a wok or large pan, cook ground turkey until browned.

2. Add vegetables and garlic, stir-fry until tender.

3. Drizzle with soy sauce and sesame oil, toss until well-coated.

Nutritional Information:

Per serving: Calories 320, Protein 25g, Fiber 5g

Amaranth Breakfast Bowl

- **Cooking Time:** 15 minutes

- **Servings:** 2

Ingredients:

- 1 cup amaranth, cooked

- 1 cup mixed berries

- 2 tablespoons Greek yogurt

- 1 tablespoon honey

- 1/4 cup sliced almonds

Instructions:

1. Cook amaranth according to package instructions.

2. Divide cooked amaranth into bowls.

3. Top with mixed berries, Greek yogurt, honey, and sliced almonds.

Nutritional Information:

Per serving: Calories 280, Protein 10g, Fiber 8g

7. Lentil and Vegetable Soup

- **Cooking Time:** 30 minutes

- **Servings:** 6

Ingredients:

- 1 cup green lentils, cooked

- 4 cups vegetable broth

- 2 cups mixed vegetables (carrots, celery, spinach)

- 1 onion, diced

- 2 cloves garlic, minced

- 1 teaspoon cumin

- Salt and pepper to taste

Instructions:

1. In a pot, sauté onion and garlic until softened.

2. Add vegetable broth, lentils, mixed vegetables, cumin, salt, and pepper.

3. Simmer for 20-25 minutes until vegetables are tender.

Nutritional Information:

Per serving: Calories 180, Protein 12g, Fiber 8g

Spinach and Feta Stuffed Chicken Breast

- **Cooking Time:** 35 minutes

- **Servings:** 2

Ingredients:

- 2 boneless, skinless chicken breasts

- 2 cups fresh spinach, chopped

- 1/4 cup feta cheese

- 1 tablespoon olive oil

- 1 teaspoon Italian seasoning

Instructions:

1. Preheat oven to 375°F (190°C).

2. In a bowl, mix chopped spinach, feta, Italian seasoning, salt, and pepper.

3. Cut a pocket in each chicken breast and stuff with the spinach mixture.

4. Drizzle olive oil over the chicken and bake for 30-35 minutes.

Nutritional Information:

Per serving: Calories 320, Protein 40g, Healthy Fats 10g

9. Broccoli and Mushroom Stir-Fry with Tofu

- **Cooking Time:** 25 minutes

- **Servings:** 4

Ingredients:

- 1 block firm tofu, cubed

- 4 cups broccoli florets

- 2 cups sliced mushrooms

- 3 tablespoons low-sodium soy sauce

- 1 tablespoon sesame oil

- 1 teaspoon ginger, minced

Instructions:

1. In a pan, stir-fry tofu until golden.

2. Add broccoli, mushrooms, and ginger, continue stirring.

3. Pour soy sauce and sesame oil over the mixture, cook until vegetables are tender.

Nutritional Information:

Per serving: Calories 250, Protein 15g, Fiber 5g

Berry Smoothie Bowl

- **Preparation Time:** 10 minutes

- **Servings:** 2

Ingredients:

- 1 cup mixed berries (strawberries, blueberries, raspberries)

- 1 banana

- 1/2 cup Greek yogurt

- 1/4 cup granola

- 1 tablespoon chia seeds

Instructions:

1. Blend mixed berries, banana, and Greek yogurt until smooth.

2. Pour into bowls and top with granola and chia seeds.

Nutritional Information:

Per serving: Calories 220, Protein 10g, Fiber 6g

BONUS CHAPTER 2

EXERCISE RECOMMENDATION

FOR BLOOD TYPE A

Maintaining a healthy and active lifestyle is essential for overall well-being, regardless of blood type. While exercise recommendations are not specifically tailored to blood types based on scientific evidence, individuals with Blood Type A may benefit from certain types of activities that align with their potential characteristics. Here are general exercise recommendations for individuals with Blood Type A:

1. Mind-Body Exercises:

- **Yoga:** Engage in yoga practices that focus on flexibility, balance, and stress reduction. Styles such as Hatha or Kundalini may be particularly beneficial.

2. Moderate Aerobic Activities:

- **Brisk Walking:** Incorporate regular brisk walking sessions into your routine. Aim for at least 30 minutes most days of the week.

- **Cycling:** Enjoy cycling at a moderate pace, whether outdoors or on a stationary bike.

3. Low-Impact Cardio Workouts:

- **Swimming:** Embrace swimming as a low-impact cardiovascular exercise that is gentle on the joints.

- **Elliptical Training:** Use an elliptical machine for a low-impact cardio workout.

4. Strength Training:

- **Bodyweight Exercises:** Include bodyweight exercises such as squats, lunges, and push-ups to build strength.

- **Pilates:** Integrate Pilates exercises to enhance core strength and improve posture.

5. Relaxation Techniques:

- **Tai Chi:** Explore the gentle, flowing movements of Tai Chi for balance, flexibility, and stress reduction.

6. Outdoor Activities:

- **Nature Walks:** Take advantage of nature walks or hikes to connect with the outdoors and promote mental well-being.

7. Consistency and Variety:

- **Consistent Routine:** Establish a consistent exercise routine that includes a mix of activities to promote overall fitness.

- **Mindful Movement:** Focus on exercises that promote mindfulness and mental clarity.

8. Individual Preferences:

- **Dance:** If you enjoy it, engage in dance as a fun and effective way to stay active.

- **Martial Arts:** Consider martial arts for a combination of physical activity and mental discipline.

9. Consultation with Health Professionals:

- **Individualized Approach:** Consult with healthcare professionals or fitness experts for personalized advice based on your health status, fitness level, and any specific considerations.

10. Listen to Your Body:

- **Intuitive Exercise:** Pay attention to how your body responds to different exercises. Choose activities that make you feel energized and invigorated.

www.ingramcontent.com/pod-product-compliance
Lightning Source LLC
Chambersburg PA
CBHW050853260726
48660CB00006B/2616